- **Book Name**

- Bodybuilding

"Anatomy of Iron:

Building the Perfect

Physique through

Bodybuilding"

- **Written by**

- Sam Berman

Table of Contents

- # "Chapter 1: Foundation of Iron."

- In "Anatomy of Iron: Building the Perfect Physique through Bodybuilding," All of the investigation into the realm of bodybuilding is laid out in this chapter by the author. The "Foundation of Iron" is a metaphor for the guiding ideas and concepts that form the basis of bodybuilding as a science and an art form.

-

  What the reader can expect to find in this first chapter is:

- The author provides an overview of the fundamental ideas and tenets that underpin bodybuilding as a sport. Topics covered may include the concepts of bodybuilding, strength training, and muscle growth.

- The chapter may stress how important it is to know one's bodily parts and how they work in relation to bodybuilding. This may shed light on the anatomical components of muscles and bones as well as the physiological mechanisms that promote muscular development.

- Tone Setting: By laying forth the book's fundamental concepts and goals, "Foundation of Iron" sets the tone for the whole thing. Its goal is to educate readers about the fundamentals of bodybuilding so that they can establish a strong foundation for their own knowledge and understanding.

- aspects of motivation: To encourage readers on their path, the chapter may contain aspects of motivation. One way to achieve this goal is to bring attention to the fact that bodybuilding has the power to improve one's physical and mental health.

- Setting the Scene: By reading this, readers may find out why certain concepts are so important while trying to achieve a certain body type. Anatomy, strength training, nutrition, and other foundational topics of bodybuilding may be laid forth in this chapter.

- Essentially, "Chapter 1: Foundation of Iron" will set the stage for the rest of the book, making sure that readers understand the basic ideas and concepts that will help them navigate the more technical aspects of bodybuilding in the chapters that follow.

• Chapter 2: The Human Machine

- In "Anatomy of Iron: Building the Perfect Physique through Bodybuilding," the second chapter, "The Human Machine," is quite important. In this chapter, the author explores the complex workings of the human body through the metaphor of a machine. In the context of bodybuilding, the name "The Human Machine" alludes to an investigation into the physiological components of the human body.

-

Some of the most important things that readers may find in this chapter are:

- Anatomy of the Human Body: This chapter probably gives an anatomy lesson, with an emphasis on the skeleton, tendons, ligaments, and connective tissues that are important for bodybuilding. Perhaps the reader will come to understand the interplay between these components and how they facilitate the growth of muscles.

- A Systematic and Organised Approach to Body Understanding: Using a machine metaphor implies a methodical and organised way to study the body. Possible topics covered include the relationship between the neurological, skeletal, and muscular systems as well as their interdependence.

- Essential Background Information for Bodybuilding: This chapter may provide readers with the necessary background information for effective bodybuilding, laying the platform for future topics. Customising exercise programmes, creating training schedules, and avoiding injuries all require an understanding of the body as a machine.

- Readers may come across real-world consequences as a result of seeing the human body through a mechanical lens. Possible topics covered include the role of correct form and technique, the relative merits of various exercises, and the best ways to train for optimum results.

- Potentially discussed in this chapter are the metabolic processes and energy needs of the body, which may provide some insight into the function that these play in the process of building muscle. When planning diets to aid in the attainment of bodybuilding objectives, this knowledge can be crucial.

- The overarching goal of "Chapter 2: The Human Machine" is to provide readers with a comprehensive view of the human body by presenting it as an intricate and ever-changing machine. Building on this foundational information, readers may apply it to their bodybuilding journey, improving their exercises and increasing the likelihood of achieving the ideal physique.

• Chapter 3: The Blueprint of Strength

- "Anatomy of Iron: Building the Perfect Physique through Bodybuilding" contains an important section titled "Chapter 3: The Blueprint of Strength." In this chapter, we will delve into the physiological aspects of strength training and how it helps achieve the larger objective of developing a defined body. A systematic investigation of the underlying concepts of strength training within the framework of bodybuilding is what "The Blueprint of Strength" alludes to.

A brief synopsis of the content that this chapter may cover is as follows:

Considerations Regarding the Body's Physiology: This chapter probably explores the body's reactions to strength training. Among the topics that might be covered are the many kinds of muscle fibres, brain adaptations, and other elements that lead to enhanced strength.

Distinct Personalities and Heredity: One critical component is elucidating the function of heredity in the maturation of strength. Possible topics covered in this chapter include the importance of individual variances in the rate and efficiency of strength development.

An explanation of the idea of progressive overload, a cornerstone of strength training, is probably in the works. In order to maintain strength gains over time, readers may discover that it is essential to progressively increase resistance or intensity.

This chapter may include practical advice on how to structure strength training programmes in order to achieve your goals. Optimal strength growth may necessitate careful consideration of exercise choice, set and rep ranges, and training frequency.

Integration with Bodybuilding Objectives: This chapter will emphasise the need of establishing strength as a basis for reaching the physique-building goals mentioned in the book, thus bridging the gap between strength training and bodybuilding.

Discussions on the importance of diet in promoting strength development may be encountered by readers. Knowledge about the significance of protein consumption, adequate hydration, and other dietary factors for achieving maximum strength gains might be included in this.

Last but not least, "Chapter 3: The Blueprint of Strength" is a blueprint for learning the fundamentals of strength training as it pertains to bodybuilding in general. This chapter gives readers the tools they need to build a powerful and defined physique by delving into the physiological foundations of strength growth and offering practical recommendations.

Chapter 4: Anatomy in Action

- The book "Anatomy of Iron: Building the Perfect Physique through Bodybuilding" contains an essential part titled "Chapter 4: Anatomy in Action." This chapter explores the intricate relationship between the human body and physical activity, highlighting the importance of knowing the biomechanics of movement for efficient bodybuilding. The title alludes to a hands-on investigation when readers discover how understanding the human body affects the performance of physical activities.
- Important things that readers may come upon in this section are:
-

  Exercise Biomechanics: This chapter probably gives a detailed breakdown of the biomechanics of a number of bodybuilding exercises. An examination of the interplay between bones, muscles, and joints is part of this.
- Proper Form and Technique: It is quite probable that the need to maintain proper form and technique during workouts will be emphasised.

By seeing the anatomy in action, readers may learn to perform motions safely and effectively, engaging their muscles to their fullest potential.

- Activation and Targeting of Muscles: Readers might learn which muscle groups are worked out in particular activities. In order to build a healthy physique and achieve certain muscle growth goals, this information is essential for creating workouts.

- The chapter can go over how important it is to mix up your workout routine to keep your muscles from getting bored and stopping growing. For long-term success, it's crucial to learn how the body responds to various motions.

- Consideration for individual differences: This may take into account things like mobility, flexibility, and anatomical variations. Readers could discover the best ways to exercise by adapting them to their own bodies.

- Injury Prevention: In order to show how a good grasp of anatomy in motion can lead to safer training techniques, it might be helpful to give practical advice for injury prevention.

- The goal of this chapter, which centres on "Anatomy in Action," is to help readers make the transition from studying anatomy in a classroom to implementing that information in a gym setting. The ideal physique described in the book is within reach, and readers will likely have a better understanding of how their bodies work during exercise as a result.

• Chapter 5: The Muscle Symphony

- An intriguing portion of "Anatomy of Iron: Building the Perfect Physique through Bodybuilding" is "Chapter 5: The Muscle Symphony." This chapter probably focuses on the significance of a balanced approach to building a body by explaining the complex relationship between various muscle groups and how they work together. The term "muscle symphony" is used metaphorically to describe the harmonious interaction of muscles that contribute to a balanced and attractive body.

-

Potential content in this chapter is as follows:

- Muscle Synergy: This chapter probably delves into the ways in which different exercises and movements include muscle synergy. The reader may come to appreciate the interplay of several muscle groups and how they work in tandem to produce power and strength.

- The achievement of balanced muscle development is the primary goal. Achieving a balanced physique where each muscle group contributes appropriately is possible, and readers may pick up some pointers on how to do just that.

- Practical guidance on targeted training to treat particular muscle groups is likely to be offered in the section on targeted training approaches. Isolation exercises, compound motions, and methods for training certain muscles to their full potential might all be part of this conversation.

- The chapter may discuss the aesthetic principles of bodybuilding, instructing readers on how to achieve aesthetically pleasing proportions. Achieving a balanced body requires knowledge of the connections between different muscle groups.

- In order to prevent imbalances and overdevelopment, readers may learn about the dangers of focusing on some muscle groups while neglecting others. Muscle imbalances can cause injuries or an unnatural look; this chapter could offer advice on how to avoid these problems.

- Personal Differences: It's possible to bring up the topic of taking into account different body types and hereditary tendencies. By understanding how to modify training methods based on one's individual physiology, readers may make the Muscle Symphony work for them.

- Emphasising "The Muscle Symphony," this chapter adds to the comprehensive comprehension of bodybuilding as an art form. The book outlines the ideal physique for its readers and encourages them to workout with care and purpose, stressing the need for coordinated muscular development.

• Chapter 6: Nutritional Foundations

- In "Anatomy of Iron: Building the Perfect Physique through Bodybuilding," the crucial "Chapter 6: Nutritional Foundations" part is located. In this chapter, the emphasis moves to the importance of nutrition in bodybuilding, specifically how a well-structured diet is the cornerstone to getting the body you want. This chapter gives the fundamentals for understanding and executing an effective nutritional strategy in the context of bodybuilding, as the title "Nutritional Foundations" suggests.

- Some of the most important things that readers may find in this chapter are:

-
The chapter probably starts out by outlining the importance of nutrition in bodybuilding and how it supports recovery, performance, and muscular growth. If readers want to know how their food

choices affect their bodybuilding objectives, they could find this article helpful.

- Proteins, carbs, and lipids, the three macronutrients, will likely be thoroughly investigated. The chapter might instruct readers on how to build their meals by discussing the precise functions of each macronutrient in energy production and muscle growth.

- Considerations Regarding Micronutrients: In addition to macronutrients, it is possible to emphasise the significance of micronutrients, which include vitamins and minerals. Potentially covered topics include the importance of certain micronutrients to general health and the effects of deficiency on physical performance.

- The chapter may explore the idea of nutritional timing, which is the idea that when you eat and what you eat affects your energy levels, muscle protein synthesis, and recovery.

- Performance and Hydration: We will most certainly talk about how staying properly hydrated helps you perform at your best during your workouts and when you recuperate. The importance of keeping one's fluid levels optimal within the framework of bodybuilding may be uncovered for readers.

- Potentially included are strategies for supplementation, which provide practical advice on how to incorporate supplements into a bodybuilding diet. Supplementing one's diet with protein, vitamins, and other nutrients may be the topic of this chapter.

- Advice on how to modify eating habits to achieve certain bodybuilding objectives, such as increasing muscle mass, decreasing body fat percentage, or keeping the weight off, may be available to readers. Considerations including metabolic rate, body composition, and training intensity could be part of this individualised strategy.

- The purpose of "Chapter 6: Nutritional Foundations" is to provide readers with the basic information they need to make educated food decisions that will help them achieve their bodybuilding goals. Readers can improve the efficacy of their workout and get closer to the ideal physique mentioned throughout the book by comprehending the nutritional principles stated in this chapter.

• "Chapter 7: Hormonal Harmony"

- There is no more important part of "Anatomy of Iron: Building the Perfect Physique through Bodybuilding" than "Chapter 7: Hormonal Harmony." This chapter probably dives into the complex web of hormones and bodybuilding, stressing how important it is to maintain a healthy hormonal balance in order to maximise muscle growth and general physical development. The title "Hormonal Harmony" implies that this chapter delves into the topic of balanced hormone function and how it relates to the bodybuilding journey.

- Important things that readers may come upon in this section are:

-

Hormonal Influences: This chapter will probably go over all the hormones that are important for bodybuilding, including growth hormone, insulin, cortisol, testosterone, and more. Muscle development, metabolic rate, and general physiological reactions are all areas that readers may learn more about thanks to these hormones.

- It is likely that there will be an emphasis on testosterone, which is frequently seen as a crucial hormone for developing muscle. The function of testosterone in establishing an anabolic state and enhancing protein synthesis in muscles is something that readers might find out.

- How Growth Hormone Aids in Recuperation: This chapter may go into detail about the role that growth hormone plays in the healing process. To get the most out of your bodybuilding efforts, it can help to know how growth hormones affect tissue repair and regeneration.

- The function of insulin in the utilisation of nutrients, especially in relation to the metabolism of carbohydrates and the synthesis of proteins, may be discussed. Insulin sensitivity and its effects on body composition could be explained to readers.

- The stress hormone cortisol may play a part in this chapter's examination of stress management by examining how levels of this hormone affect muscular breakdown and repair. We may talk about ways to control our stress and cortisol levels.

- Insights into the ways in which exercise, particularly resistance training, affects hormone reactions may be available to readers. Training methods can be fine-tuned for maximum effect by studying the hormonal adaptations to various forms of exercise.

- Natural Hormone Balancing: Maybe you'll find some helpful tips on how to improve your lifestyle by paying more attention to things like sleep, food, and stress management. Holistic living choices can help readers achieve hormonal equilibrium.

- Emphasising "hormonal harmony," this chapter seeks to educate readers on the intricate relationship between hormones and bodybuilding. In order to maximise training and attain the ideal physique described in the book, readers should familiarise themselves with the ways in which hormones react to different stimuli and the effects of lifestyle choices on hormonal balance.

Chapter 8: Recovery and Regeneration

- In "Anatomy of Iron: Building the Perfect Physique through Bodybuilding," the eighth chapter, "Recovery and Regeneration," is an essential component. The importance of recovery and regeneration in maximising muscle growth, performance, and general health is likely to be discussed in this chapter. The focus, as implied by the title, is on the mechanisms that enable the body to regenerate and recover after strenuous training in order to face future difficulties.

- Some of the most important things that readers may find in this chapter are:

-

You should expect this chapter to stress how crucial recovery is to your bodybuilding quest. While we sleep, our bodies mend and strengthen themselves, and maybe that makes more sense to readers.

- Strategies for Muscle Healing: This section may offer useful advice on how to speed up the process of muscle healing. Possible topics covered include what to eat and drink after an exercise, how to employ recovery techniques like foam rolling and massage, and how much water to drink.

- Sleep and Regeneration: The significance of sleep for healing will most certainly be front and centre. The significance of getting a good night's sleep for regulating hormones, repairing muscles, and maintaining general health may be revealed to readers.

- Recovery tactics: active and passive This chapter may differentiate between recovery tactics that are active and those that are passive. Light workouts or other low-intensity activities may be part of an active recovery plan, while relaxation and rest may be the focus of a passive recovery plan. It would be easy for readers to implement each strategy in their daily lives.

- Diet for Recovery: It's possible to incorporate an in-depth analysis of the role that diet plays in the healing process. To aid with muscle glycogen replenishment and protein synthesis, this may include talking about when and what to eat.

- Injury Prevention and Rehabilitation: Realistic suggestions for avoiding injuries and developing plans to recover from them may be covered. The significance of a good warm-up, cool-down, and workouts to increase flexibility and joint health could be enlightened to the readers.

- Connection Between Mental Health and Rehabilitation: This chapter may go into detail about how mental health relates to rehabilitation. We might look at ways to keep a good outlook, practice mindfulness, and deal with stress.

- Readers may come across articles discussing periodization, a training cycle planning technique that incorporates both high- and low-intensity intervals. Adequate recovery and the avoidance of burnout are both made possible by this methodically planned strategy.

- The goal of this chapter, which centres on "Recovery and Regeneration," is to provide readers with the information they need to develop effective recovery plans. Learning how to properly support the body while it rests improves training efficacy and gets readers one step closer to the ideal physique described in the book as a whole.

• Chapter 9: Mind-Muscle Connection

- "Chapter 9: Mind-Muscle Connection" explores the mental side of bodybuilding, highlighting the significance of maintaining a solid rapport between one's thoughts and the muscles they are working. This chapter probably delves into the ways that being mentally present, focused, and purposeful during exercises can lead to better muscle engagement, growth, and success in bodybuilding as a whole. In the context of developing an ideal body, the title "Mind-Muscle Connection" implies that this section explores the deep connection between one's mental states and their physical performance.

- Some of the most important things that readers may find in this chapter are:

-

The chapter will probably define and clarify the notion of the mind-muscle connection, which is essential for understanding the relationship between the two. By paying close attention and focusing their minds, readers may be able to get the most out of every repetition and exercise.

- advise on visualisation approaches: This section could contain practical advice on visualisation approaches. In this article, readers will discover how to visualise the muscle group being worked in order to increase the quality of their workouts by recruiting more muscle fibres.

- The significance of maintaining attention and concentration throughout exercise is likely to be emphasised. Muscle engagement and general growth might be impeded by distractions and a lack of focus, which may be addressed in the chapter.

- During training, readers may come across discussions about how deliberate each movement is. Being completely engaged in the activity requires bringing one's attention to the here and now and deliberately tensing and releasing muscles.

- The practice of mindful movement, in which one is completely present with one's bodily feelings and motions, is one such idea that may be investigated. The mind-muscle connection and training results can be improved with this mindful method.

- Overcoming Training Plateaus: We may talk about ways to break through training plateaus by strengthening the link between the mind and the muscles. In order to revitalise development, it may be necessary to make adjustments to training methods, pay more attention to form, or add new exercises.

- Increased motivation, a feeling of empowerment, and a more positive attitude towards training are some of the psychological benefits of a strong mind-muscle connection that may be discussed in the chapter.

- There may be examples and explanations of how to apply the mind-muscle link to different types of workouts. Potentially useful for readers are explanations of how to implement these concepts in compound and isolation movements.

- Emphasising the "Mind-Muscle Connection," this chapter seeks to demonstrate how incorporating mental focus and intentionality into one's bodybuilding regimen may yield remarkable results. Gaining a deeper understanding of the mind-muscle link and learning to control it can make training more enjoyable and productive, leading readers closer to the ideal body type addressed throughout the book.

• Chapter 10: The Perfect Physique

- Building the Perfect Physique through Bodybuilding concludes with "Chapter 10: The Perfect Physique" in "Anatomy of Iron." This last chapter gives readers a rundown of the fundamentals and some pointers on how to make their own unique bodybuilding programme. Based on the title, it seems like this chapter is going to compile all the information from the others into a detailed plan for getting the body you want.

- In this final chapter, readers may come across the following important elements:

-

The chapter will probably start out by restating the basic ideas that have been covered in the book so far. The purpose of this summary is to restate the main ideas so that readers fully grasp the fundamentals of effective bodybuilding.

- Concept Integration: This chapter could centre on bringing together several ideas, such as anatomy, strength training, nutrition, and recovery. The reader is likely to observe the integrated nature of these components as they pertain to bodybuilding.

- Customisation: You can expect to receive useful guidance on how to design a unique bodybuilding programme. By taking into account each reader's unique objectives, dietary preferences, and physiological reactions, the author may suggest ways to improve training, nutrition, and recovery.

- Achievable and Realistic Goal Setting: This chapter could stress the significance of goal setting. In order to achieve their intended physical results, readers may find it helpful to create SMART goals—goals that are clear, measurable, and have a deadline.

- Sustainability in the Long Run: We May Talk About How to Keep Your Bodybuilding Progress Going Strong Over the Long Run. Some possible approaches to this problem include being adaptable, keeping oneself motivated, and avoiding burnout.

- Tools and methods for keeping tabs on development might be incorporated. By keeping tabs on their progress in key areas like strength and muscle mass, readers can make sure they're heading in the correct direction.

- Adaptability and Flexibility: This chapter might stress how crucial it is to be able to change and adjust as you progress through your bodybuilding adventure. Readers may find helpful advice on how to adapt their plans to new information, personal tastes, or developing objectives.

- Honouring Accomplishments: It is probable that you will receive encouragement to honour accomplishments, regardless of their size. A good outlook and ongoing motivation can be enhanced by acknowledging accomplishments and stepping stones along the way.

- Embracing the Journey: In the last chapter, the author may suggest that readers view bodybuilding as an ongoing quest for personal growth. Learning, growing, and relishing in the transforming experience could be emphasised.

- With an emphasis on "The Perfect Physique," this last chapter seeks to offer readers a guide for putting theoretical understanding into practice. In it, the author lays out the fundamentals of bodybuilding and provides readers with the information they need to start their own personal path towards their ideal physique.